TEN STEPS TO DETOX YOU

DETOX YOUR BODY AND FEEL REJUVINATED

including

TEMPLATE FOR YOUR LIFE PLAN

NATASHA DAVIS

TEN STEPS TO DETOX YOU. DETOX YOUR BODY AND FEEL REJUVINATED including TEMPLATE FOR YOUR LIFE PLAN

On Instagram as natashahubczenkodavis

Published in Melbourne, Australia.

FIRST EDITION

ISBN 978-1-09-995472-6

ABOUT THE AUTHOR
NATASHA DAVIS

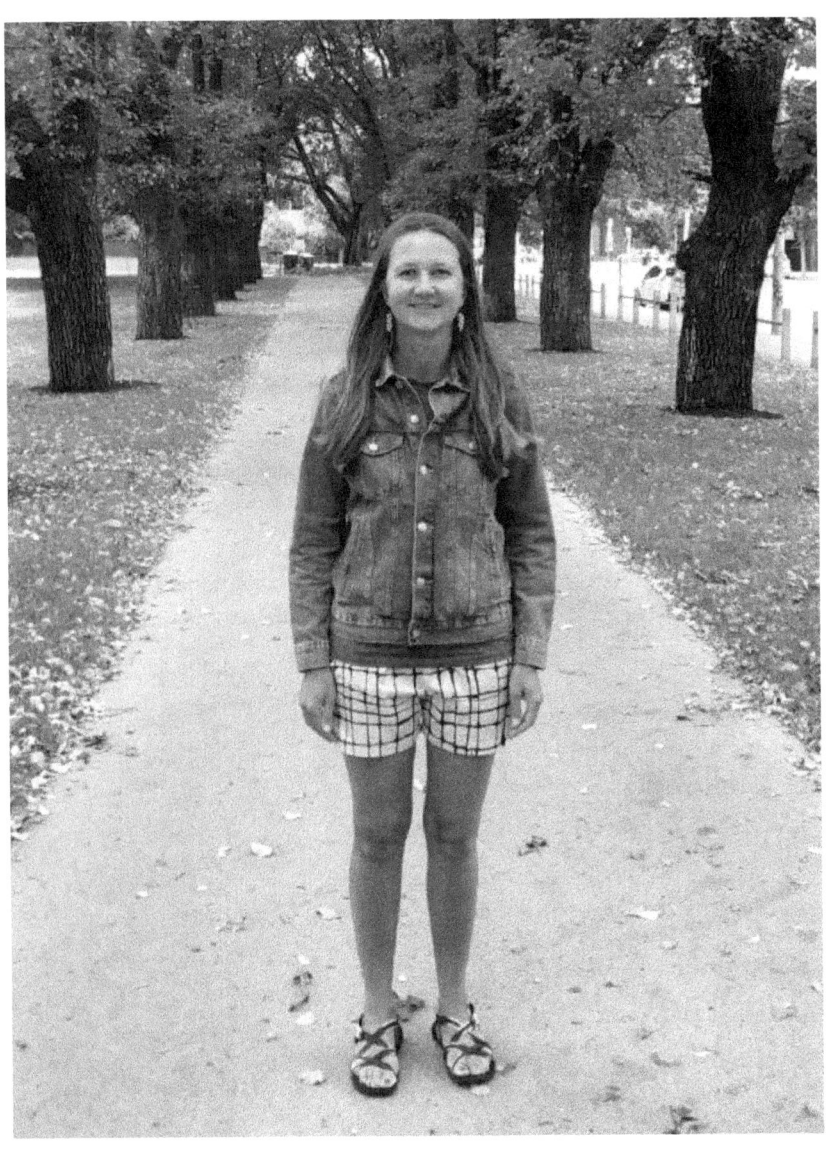

NATASHA DAVIS developed this book through life hacks she conducted on herself to achieve and maintain health, while living and working in the heavily populated, urbanized Asian city, Manila, Philippines, over the past eighteen years, and travelling internationally extensively. Through these experiences, she has been able to witness health remedies and wellness routines used throughout the world, and she has learnt that good health is not related to a person's income, or the wealth of the country they live in. She believes that good health and wellness should happen for you, without making any concerted effort by living in harmony with your environment.

The author now lives in Australia with her family which includes children born, and with their teenage years lived in Manila, Philippines. Growing up children in a mega city in Asia provides its own challenges in relation to: food availability, food quality, food hygiene, water and air quality due to pollution, bacteria, viruses, fungi, heavy metals, and chemicals.

The world's water and air are now heavily polluted. The soils relied on for food are nutrient deficient, and polluted. To remain healthy requires effort, and the starting point for good health is an excellent detoxification system.

TEN STEPS TO DETOX YOU, Detox Your Body And Feel Rejuvenated, is an easy to follow guide for your achievement of better, day to day health.

To help in organizing your thoughts on what is important to you, and how best to prioritize your time over five years, the author developed and included the 'Template For Your Life Plan'.

CONTENTS

INTRODUCTION

I like most people have previously lived a life surrounded by chemicals in cleaning products, hair dye, makeup, and topical skin products. Consumed food with artificial colors, flavors, and preservatives, contaminated with pesticides, heavy metals and bacteria, and genetically modified. Consumed water that is overly processed, contaminated with bacteria and heavy metals. Swam in chlorinated swimming pools, and stagnant lakes. Taken the doctor's prescriptions for antibiotics and pain medicines, so that I stayed in office instead of taking sick days, and working long hours.

I add to this, breathing in heavily polluted air, both indoors and outdoors; and living in a highly populated, high density city with high humidity, and rainfall. Brought me to be exposed to many different types of antibiotic resistant bacteria, parasites, viruses, fungi, heavy metals and chemicals.

What does it take to feel healthy every day?

Has good health eluded you, all your life, and you don't know where to start?

Do you feel that your living environment is bringing your health markers down?

Do you feel that your life habits are not optimal?

Do you know where you are going in the next five years of your life?

Your health experiences many challenges due to food availability, quality, hygiene, nutrient deficiencies, food and drinking water contamination with heavy metals and chemicals, drinking water shortages, poor quality outdoor and indoor air due to pollution, and air borne bacteria, viruses, fungi, heavy metals and chemicals.

It can be difficult to know what path to follow in living a healthy life. There is a barrage of advertising that sells the lifestyle, and health benefits of consuming products that may contain chemicals, heavy metals, and bacteria promising that you will feel better for it.

I favour the use of natural therapies and approaches, to avoid, and solve health concerns, but of course if a major emergency occurred then I would go to the hospital for treatment. I have lived and worked in the Asian city, Manila, Philippines for 18 years. I travelled extensively internationally, and now reside again in Australia. I have had the opportunity in my life to meet with many people of different cultures, and with this I have learnt about differing philosophies to living and health management. From people who have diets much worse than my own ever was, that are based around fast and packaged food, and inactive lifestyles. As well as from people with lifestyles based around spiritual awareness and increasing self-knowledge.

CHAPTER ONE

ADVISORY

I am a non-medical practitioner who has performed life hacks on myself for the purpose of having the most super charged immune system, and to achieve a healthy life. I lived, and worked for 18 years in the highly populated, high density, humidity and rainfall, city of Manila, Philippines.

Always consult your medical practitioner for formal advice if you have a serious medical condition. Do not undertake the detox program if you are pregnant, or are under the age of 18 years old.

NATASHA DAVIS

CHAPTER TWO

DETOX REASON

Ageing is merely the lessening of our bodies ability to effectively detox to remove our end of life cells, and to regenerate our cells in the blood, organs, muscles, and lymphatic system. Every day we are exposed to contaminants and toxins in the air breathed in outdoors, and in the office, and homes from the furniture, wall, ceiling, and floor claddings, through the water and food consumed, through the topical application of products, and the water bathed in.

These contaminants and toxins are bacteria, parasites, fungi, heavy metals, and chemicals. They will harm you if they are not eliminated through the skin, bowels, or urine, and they will accumulate where-ever they can in your cells, blood, organs, muscles, and lymphatic system.

All live contaminants accumulated in your body need to be fed, and they like what you eat. They will feed before you do, and these contaminants expel waste toxins that cause you to feel unwell, give you aches and pains, stimulate your body to fight internal inflammation, wearing out your body quicker, and accelerating aging. Should you have a deficiency in your body of a particular mineral then another mineral may substitute, but this mineral would most likely be toxic.

Your ability to effectively detox is also affected by the energy vibrations of the people, and environment around you. Negative energy comes from pollution, negative people, built in environments without open spaces, environments without trees, flowers, birds and other wildlife, environments without clear sunlight, and environments without clean bodies of water such as rivers, oceans, and mountain fed lakes.

5

It is possible to reverse the ageing in your body inflicted through circumstances of life, and lifestyle choices as the human body has an amazing ability to heal itself, and to regenerate.

The sooner you start your detoxification journey, the better. Your goal is to initially slow, and then to halt the progression of ageing, so that your quality of life can improve through your ability to do more for yourself, and to lessen your aches and pain. As your body detoxifies further with time, you can experience a feeling of health that for some people they have never had, and for others a feeling of health they only experienced during childhood, and teenage years.

CHAPTER THREE

DETOX COMMITMENT

The process of detoxification is not easy, and at times it can be painful, as you can feel worse than you did before you started due to the physical, and emotional process of your body releasing stored contaminants and toxins.

You will ask yourself how did I get myself into this mess?

You need to be committed to your detoxification, and keep in mind your goal for the achievement of a meaningful life. A two-year commitment is needed to reverse the worst of the damage caused by disease, medicines, extreme lifestyle habits like over-exercising and substance abuse, and the circumstances of life. Over time good habits will replace your bad habits, and the process of detoxification will become easier for you.

Are you ready? You are for sure, because getting old is not your age but how many years you have left to live. Detoxification can prolong your life end date, and give you better overall health.

'The Detox Commitment is that I am worthy, and I make a commitment to myself to treat my body, mind, and soul with utmost respect. I heal all past physical, emotional, and spiritual damage that I, and others have inflicted upon me.'

CHAPTER FOUR

TEN STEPS TO DETOX YOU SYSTEM

The TEN STEPS TO DETOX YOU is a system to detox your body so you feel rejuvenated. The ten steps that you will move through are:

1. Self-Assessment
2. Digestive System and Food
3. Water
4. Elimination of Toxins
5. Essential Oils
6. Pure Fruit Syrups, Herbal and Botanical Tonics
7. Charcoal
8. Iodine and Colloidal Silver
9. Reassess Your Friendship Circle and Hobbies
10. Reassess Your Financial Outflows and Time-Consuming Responsibilities

CHAPTER FIVE

DETOX STEP 1: SELF–ASSESSMENT

L et's get started on your self-assessment of the TEN STEPS TO DETOX YOU – Detox Your Body And Feel Rejuvenated – Step One.

Start with making a self-assessment list of your daily life routines and state, under the headings of health, food, water, light, move your body, sleep, social interactions, and self-expression. The self-assessment list has two columns: pros and cons.

HEALTH
How do you feel every day?
Do you have brain fog, aches, pains, or more complicated health issues?
Good health is the foundation in your life and is worth being your primary focus, and time investment.
You will need to write down all your symptoms and conditions. Here is your check list of possible, but not complete symptoms and conditions:

- food allergies
- itchy skin
- jaundice
- constipation
- irritable bowel syndrome
- parasites
- acid reflux
- small intestine bacterial growth
- digestion problems

11

- high or low blood pressure
- diabetes
- lung problems
- heart problems
- immune system problems
- urinary tract and kidney problems
- reproductive organ problems
- cancer
- ulcers
- anemia
- bloated stomach
- headache
- fluid retention
- joint and muscle pains
- neurological problems
- sinusitis
- thyroid problems

FOOD

Food can be contaminated with bacteria, parasites, pesticides and other chemicals, heavy metals, antibiotics, and can also include artificial colors and flavors, and preservatives. It is important to know your food country of origin as a minimum, and as much about the food growing, production and hygiene handling processes of the farmer, manufacturer, distribution chain, and retailer. Poor and unsanitary food growing practices in relation to fertilization and watering of vegetables, fruits and crops, unsanitary animal husbandry practices, and a lack of refrigeration of the food introduces contaminants that are toxic for you. A good practice is to buy local produce, direct from the farm, or at farmers markets, and buying organic if available, and affordable.

You need to reduce your consumption of sugar, and heavily processed vegetable oils. Natural oils such as coconut, olive, and avocado oil are good for you. Your body needs some salt to balance your electrolytes, but it should be taken in moderation. Spices and herbs are good for your health.

Read the ingredients list on prepared, and packaged food that you buy to make sure that you are getting more nutrition per gram consumed than sugar, oil, and bulking products such as soy. If you are buying a burger made of a protein from the retailer, then read the ingredients list and select the product with more protein, a low amount of filler product, little or no preservatives, and no artificial colors and flavors. It is better still to buy and consume your protein on the same day, as refrigeration practices at the retailer may not be optimum, and the shelf life can be overestimated resulting in the food rotting before the listed expiry date.

Packaged and canned foods can have a high sugar and salt content, artificial colors, flavors and preservative and these are bad for your health, so eat sparingly. You can achieve better health outcomes with fresh foods, if they are available. If you buy canned foods, be aware that the lining of the can may have the toxin bisphenol-A (BPA). Don't buy a can of food that is dented, and don't store an open can of food in the refrigerator.

Do you not know how to cook?
Do you have time constraints?
Do you have a lack of interest in cooking?
Are you buying your food mostly at?
- restaurants
- as take-out
- from the prepared meal frozen section of the supermarket

It would be a good idea to learn some cooking basics.

Step one, is to go to the food retailer and select the ingredients yourself for your pantry.

Step two, is to make your meal preparation really simple.

Step three, is to eat a big meal when you can. You can reduce the number of your main meals down from three, to two, by eating a big breakfast and a big dinner, or alternatively a light and easily prepared breakfast, followed by a large lunch, and a light dinner.

For breakfast you can try cooked eggs, ham, rice, and cucumber; cooked fish and vegetables; porridge of cooked oats; homemade toasted muesli; fruits, cheese, bread, sliced meats and fish. For lunch and dinner, one pot cooking that includes onion, other vegetables, and protein saves a lot of cooking, and pot cleaning time. This meal can be accompanied with bread, rice, or potato as a side dish. Pasta as a main meal provides too much sugar into the blood stream at one time, and is best eaten in small portions as a side dish.

The benefit of cooking your own meals include knowing exactly what ingredients are used, and being able to go lighter on the sugar, salt, oil added, because using more of these items is the simplest method to make food tastier, but less healthy for you.

Your budget will also improve because your cost outlay for food expenses decreases.

Buy in season, or grow your own vegetables and fruits. Buy a good quality cooking oil of olive, coconut or avocado; natural sea salt with iodine; spices and herbs; and brown or coconut sugar. The bread with mixed whole grains and seeds is the best type, if your digestive system can manage. Grains and seeds, including oats, rice, wheat, and others, need to be clean of pesticides and fertilizers and not stored in a silo or shed for many years before use, as they can become contaminated with mold, rodents, and birds.

Buy proteins that are clean, freshly prepared, and with good refrigeration or ice packing, otherwise go to the fresh produce market very early in the morning. Use your taste buds for quality control. If the food tastes bad, it is likely to be contaminated, and you should stop eating immediately. Gravies and sauces can be used to cover the taste of contaminated cheese and other proteins, and sometimes chemicals are used by food sellers to hide the visibility of bacteria in the food.

WATER
You should drink enough water so you are not dehydrated or bloated. If you are experiencing headaches the cause could be dehydration or an electrolyte imbalance. If you live in an environment where water quality is poor, installing an on-tap reverse osmosis filtration system will provide you with health benefits, and they are available from the hardware store. This is better than drinking tap water of questionable quality or bought water that may, or may not be properly filtered and sanitized.

LIGHT
Wake when the sun rises and don't keep resetting the alarm clock for another five minutes sleep before you get out of bed. If you feel tired, then go to bed and don't stay up watching television, on the computer, tablet, or handheld telephone. Try to wake, and go to sleep

at the same time everyday as this sets your internal time clock making it easier for you to manage your sleep patterns.

MOVE YOUR BODY

Light exercises that stretch and strengthen your body, and those that use your own body weight are essential for the achievement of good health. The objective in moving your body is to achieve a strong structural frame which includes having flexible and strong muscles, ligaments, and tendons. This builds resiliency in your body so that you are less susceptible to permanent injury should you fall over.

Often when using indoor gym equipment, the objective is to build the large muscles in the body, but this approach can weaken your tendons and ligaments, making you vulnerable to injury that take a long time to heal.

Exercise through every day movements, such as walking to your activities, biking, using public transport, walking to the grocery store, carrying the groceries home, cleaning your home, gardening, cooking your meals, hanging your laundry outside, yoga, gymnastics, playing sport, walking the stairs etc. If you have time, joining in a team sport provides exercise and social interactions that give you a better understanding of yourself, and others.

SLEEP

For a more restful sleep, make sure your environment is dark, low noise, and cool. It is worth investing in good quality bedding, as about eight hours of sleep is recommended. This means you spend at least one third of each day sleeping.

SOCIAL INTERACTIONS

Make time for social interactions, and they can be as simple as engaging with people as you go about your everyday activities. From these interactions you will learn more about yourself, and what is important to you, plus you will gain a better appreciation of what is important to other people.

The key is not to compete with other people through words, and boasting on fashion, sports, education, achievements, and ownership of things. Compete with only yourself.

Determine how good you really are at something by setting yourself time-based performance targets, and conduct your own assessment to determine your level of achievement and areas for improvement.

You don't need other people telling you that you are good or bad, because this is coming from their biased perspective. Also, don't get down if you don't achieve your performance target as the target could have been too aggressive and/or the actions not the right ones, or you were never really interested in this performance target so it was the wrong one for you.

SELF-EXPRESSION

People are designed to self-express themselves through their clothing, hairstyle, opinions, and lifestyle choices.

Attempting to conform to others' opinions obtained from the media or shared with you by a friend, social group, office colleague, or family will cause a disconnect between your version of yourself, and this imposed version. This results in your personal misery and poor health as it is not possible to conform to this false reality, and their need to control you.

The key here is to understand that these are other people's problems and not yours, that you don't need to internalize other people's problems and accept their deconstruction of your self-esteem.

Sometimes you have to realize that you can't help people who don't want to help themselves, as their intention is to cause others' harm. It is best to put some distance between them and you.

CHAPTER SIX

DETOX STEP 2: DIGESTIVE SYSTEM AND FOOD

L et's review your digestive system and food of the TEN STEPS TO DETOX YOU – Detox Your Body And Feel Rejuvenated – Step Two.

The digestive system encompasses the esophagus, stomach, small and large intestines, appendix, gallbladder, liver, pancreas, and mouth/saliva.

Do you suffer from constipation, irritable bowel syndrome or both?
Do you have autoimmune issues such as itchy skin or lupus?
Is your blood sugar level out of control, or in control but with an upwards trajectory?
Do you have acid reflux and heart burn?
Do you have allergies to food and/or the environment?

DIGESTIVE SYSTEM OVERLOADED
To start detoxing your digestive system you need to first simplify your diet, and to consume a lower volume of food and beverages. Too much consumption variety confuses the digestive system, and increases the possibility that you have eaten contaminated food. Too much volume consumption makes it difficult for your digestive system to break down the food and beverages, and to use the nutrients in your body.

In a poorly functioning digestive system, your stomach acid has weakened and your blood cleaning organs such as the liver, gallbladder, kidneys, and spleen are congested and are not functioning optimally. It might be that the problem started in your stomach, or that it started in one of your organs, and the result is overall poor digestion, with pain in the digestive system.

Your body can't keep the contaminants and toxins generated from bacteria, parasites, viruses, fungi, heavy metals and chemicals to a low level. These contaminants and toxins recirculate within you, and the bacteria, parasites, viruses, and fungi increase rapidly in number colonizing you. The walls of your intestines are compromised and leak protein particles, contaminants, and toxins into your blood stream causing an immune response, and allergies.

SIMPLIFY YOUR DIET

Initially you will need to avoid grains with gluten, dairy, and high glycemic index fruits (high sugar content in relation to the water and fiber content).

You should eat mostly vegetables, fish, chicken, and eggs. Hard cheese can be eaten in moderation, if this is your main protein source, but soft cheeses should be excluded from your diet. The vegetables and proteins need to be cooked to eliminate any bacteria, and for easier digestion. Avoid deep fried food. Sweet potato is an easy to digest carbohydrate source. A small amount of white rice can be consumed as it is easy to digest and gluten free. Green shakes can provide your body with the nutrients from raw salad vegetables. Take a high-quality coconut oil directly as a tablespoon at a time, and cook your foods in coconut, olive, or avocado oil. All desserts, including ice-cream, and candy are to be avoided. Dark chocolate of a high cocoa grade can help fill most sugar cravings.

Eliminate all soft drinks, fruit shakes and fruit juices. Drink lots of pure water including mineral water, but you should feel neither dehydrated or bloated. Check the pH of your water to make sure that it is either neutral or alkaline. Start your day with two glasses of water. Herbal teas can be beneficial for healing your body. Coffee should be avoided initially, as it is acidic in pH, but if you need it, then just have it.

ANTI-PARASITIC TREATMENT

Parasites are live organisms and they can live in your blood, organs, muscles, lymphatic fluid and your digestive system. They need to be fed, taking nutrition out of your body, and excreting waste that your body will have an immune response to.

If your stomach acid is weak, then your immune system function is low in ability, and this makes you more susceptible to picking up parasites through your digestive system from food and water.

Take a natural anti-parasitic, and take it repeatedly over about six months, especially if you have spent a lot of time in outdoor activities such as swimming, and camping, and living in environments where the food or water supply is likely to be contaminated.

Your pets should also be given a natural anti-parasitic treatment.

NUTRIENT DEFICIENCIES

If you have digestive issues, it is highly likely that your absorption of nutrients is low, resulting in anemia and other mineral deficiencies. Be patient, your digestive system needs to heal itself slowly, find its balance, and these conditions will slowly disappear. If you try to rush this process, the consequence is too much detoxification an overloaded liver, kidneys and spleen, the cleansers of toxins in your body, and there will be recirculation and reabsorption of these toxins in your blood and organs.

VITAMIN D

Natural sunlight exposure on the skin stimulates your body to produce vitamin D. You should have your vitamin D levels checked, and try to spend time in the direct sunlight without sunscreen, and without getting burnt, or reddening your skin. Sunlight is an excellent sanitizer for your skin, clothing, towels, and bedding.

SLEEP

Your body performs a large number of health, and healing fixes while you are sleeping. Eight hours of sleep is usually sufficient, but if you are younger you may need more hours to accommodate the growth of your body.

PHARMACEUTICALS

Should you be taking more than one pharmaceutical medicine at any point in time, it is important to be aware that medicines interact with each other, and that medical clinical trials do not take into consideration how a particular medicine will function in the body if a person is also taking medicine A, B and C. Apply the same rationalization when taking natural medicines. You want to be certain that whatever you are taking internally is giving you an improvement in health, and equally is not detrimental to you.

CHAPTER SEVEN

DETOX STEP 3: WATER

L et's review your water of the TEN STEPS TO DETOX YOU – Detox Your Body And Feel Rejuvenated – Step Three.

You can't assume that the water that comes into your home and office provided by the government authority is of drinking quality, as it could be contaminated with bacteria, parasites, heavy metals, and chemicals. The water source and the water purification plant are usually a large distance from your home and office, and the water is distributed through a network of mains and local distribution pipes, including those inside homes, office buildings, and associated outdoor areas. The pipes of the water distribution system may be made of toxic material, have rust and breaks, and have a toxic material lining or sealant. The water source maybe contaminated due to low rainfall, resulting in the poor replenishment of the dams and aquifers.

Boiling water will kill bacteria and parasites, but this won't remove the heavy metals and chemicals making it unsafe to drink. Some of these heavy metals occur naturally in the rocks, and others are from the water distribution network. The chemicals in the drinking water may not have been removed during the filtration process. The water could have unacceptable levels of arsenic, mercury, lead, fluoride, chlorine, pharmaceuticals, pesticides, PCBs (polychlorinated biphenyls), DDT (dichloro-diphenyl-trichloroethane), fuel additives, and many other chemicals.

Check the reputation of the water supplier company if you are buying water in bottles, or tanked to your home. The water maybe contaminated, and improperly filtered. Unless otherwise specified, filtered water will generally be acidic in pH as the key minerals of calcium and magnesium have also been removed.

To have a successful detoxification journey, you need to drink plenty of water that is clean of contaminants and toxins, and is mineralized as your kidneys need water to clear out the toxic substances in your blood for disposal as urine.

DRINKING WATER
So, what can you do?

One option is to drink mineralized water from a natural spring source that has the reputation as reliable, and clean.

Another option is to install a reverse osmosis water filtration system on your tap outlet where the water source is from a rain-water tank, river stream, or the commercially provided water system. The reverse osmosis water filtration system is inexpensive in comparison to the illnesses that can result from drinking contaminated water, or water with an acidic pH. These water filtration systems are conveniently available in hardware stores and specialist providers.

As you are in charge of the maintenance of the reverse osmosis water filtration system, you can be confident that the water is clean, and this may not be the case when purchasing filtered bottled water as your water supply.

Also, some reverse osmosis water filtration systems add in alkalizing minerals of calcium and magnesium, and these electrolytes are essential for the optimal functioning of the body.

SALT WATER
Swimming in the ocean is a good way to relax, and to detox not only your skin, but also your mucous membranes, as the benefits come from both the salt and the pH of the water. If you don't like swimming, then inhaling salty, sea air by spending time at the seaside will be valuable in improving your health.

Drinking a small amount of iodized table salt (preferably a naturally evaporated sea salt) dissolved in warm water can help in balancing your electrolytes in the body as it contains sodium chloride, and the iodine is beneficial for the thyroid. An additional benefit is that the need to wake up in the middle of the night to urinate may also be reduced.

EPSON SALT BATH (MAGNESIUM SULFATE)

Bathing in warm Epson salts can relax your body, providing magnesium through your skin. Magnesium is needed by your body in many biochemical reactions, and is an electrolyte.

CHAPTER EIGHT

DETOX STEP 4: ELIMINATION OF TOXINS

Let's review the elimination of toxins in the TEN STEPS TO DETOX YOU – Detox Your Body And Feel Rejuvenated – Step Four.

The human body systems involved in the elimination of contaminants, and toxins are the digestive, circulatory, lymphatic, respiratory, and urinary systems. These systems need to be in good working order for you to experience good health.

Your body will try to break down, and eliminate any bacteria, parasites, viruses, fungi, heavy metals and chemicals that you come into contact with through ingestion, your nasal passages, skin, and eyes. If these contaminants are not eliminated, over time the accumulation slows down the functioning of your body, including the renewal of the cells and blood, which can lead to the growth of tumors, and some could be cancerous.

If your body systems are not operating optimally, or the extent of the contamination is high, then your body systems will coat these contaminants and toxins with a mineral, or another substance to quarantine you, from them, storing them in your blood, lymphatic fluid, organs, and muscles.

DIGESTIVE SYSTEM: LIVER AND GALLBLADDER

In Detox Step 2: Digestive System and Food, the role your diet, and good digestion contributes to your health is explained. The liver is a very important organ in cleaning your blood, making nutrients available, creating the bile your stomach needs to make gastric acid for the breakdown of food. The liver can get congested with gallbladder, and liver stones that form around a solid nucleus contaminant. Gallbladder stones interfere with the body's ability to release bile, and liver stones affect the body's ability to detoxify. This means that the ability to rid yourself of contaminants and toxins is poor, and they will recirculate within you, creating a virtuous circle of contamination.

If you do not have a system in place for removing these gallbladder stones naturally, they will continue to grow in size and harden. In many instances, surgical procedures have been used to remove gallbladders, and medical/surgical procedures to remove gallbladder stones.

There are two options to detox the gallbladder and the liver. One option is to fast over the course of a day, in the evening drink a glass or two of warm diluted apple cider vinegar or lemon juice, to be followed by a few tablespoons of olive oil. Then lie down on your left side for at least a couple of hours, or for the night time sleep with a heat pack (if you have one) placed on your right side, where your liver and gallbladder are located. Try to relax as the gallbladder and liver stones are released. Another option is to fast over the course of a day, in the evening take one tablespoon of Epson salt in a glass of warm water, and lie down on your left side for the night time sleep. The heat pack is optional, but it does reduce the pain due to the release of the gallbladder and liver stones. Do not do both detox options on the same night, but do monitor the results. Repeat this detox as often as you need, to improve the functioning of these organs.

CIRCULATORY SYSTEM
To improve blood circulation throughout the body through the dilation of blood vessels, vaporize and inhale cinnamon essential oil, which also has anti-bacterial properties.

Other options for improving blood circulation include, high intensity exercise or hot sauna, where the body heats up, and your perspiration aids the detoxification.

LYMPHATIC SYSTEM AND IMMUNE SYSTEM
A different approach is needed to detoxify the lymphatic system, spleen, thyroid, adrenals that are part of your immune system. They respond well to bitter foods and bitter tonics such as Swedish Bitters

and herbs, as they stimulate the organs and the digestive system kick starting the decongestion.

The lymphatic system can have blockages, and congestion. Cells in your body have a life and death cycle, and a poorly performing lymphatic system will not remove the dead cells. These end of life cells will grow, clump together to become a benign, or malignant tumor.

The human body needs movement to push oxygen throughout it, also, for the elimination of waste stored in all organs including the circulatory, lymphatic, respiratory, and urinary systems.

It is critical to have an excellent functioning lymphatic system and jumping, skipping, running, bouncing can help move your lymphatic fluids. Other options include, body massage, or a hot steam bath to open the pores in the skin and encourage perspiration.

Lemon essential oil has anti-bacterial properties, and can improve the flow of your lymphatic fluids when vaporized and inhaled.

RESPIRATORY SYSTEM

The lungs and sinuses can become congested, resulting in breathing issues, and allergic reactions. The vaporization and inhalation of essential oils with anti-bacterial, viral, and fungal properties can provide relief. Some suggestions are lavender, cinnamon, oregano, hyssop, clove, lemon, lemon grass, and tea tree oil.

Other options include, breathing in the salt air from the ocean, and swimming in the ocean as saline solutions have disinfecting properties. Mountain areas, especially those with forests of pine trees can help improve your breathing. Geothermal hot mineral springs can be consumed, bathed in, and the vapors inhaled for relief with respiratory congestions and other ailments.

URINARY SYSTEM

For your kidneys and bladder, drink plenty of water and make sure your electrolytes are in balance.

Do not drink sports drinks with high sugar content. An electrolyte powder for rehydration from gastrointestinal issues will do the same for you.

To cleanse your kidneys of stones, use the same detoxification regime for the liver and gallbladder cleanse of fasting until evening, and then consuming a glass or two of warm diluted apple cider vinegar or lemon juice, followed by consuming a few tablespoons of olive oil, and taking rest for several hours laying on your left side.

CHAPTER NINE

DETOX STEP 5: ESSENTIAL OILS

How to use essential oils of the TEN STEPS TO DETOX YOU – Detox Your Body And Feel Rejuvenated – Step Five.

Natural healthy holistic living and using what is available in your environment as a tonic is easy to do. Many pharmaceuticals are designed to replicate what was already available in nature, including those found in the rainforests, but are synthetic.

The human body is contiguous, and this means that what you breathe in, and consume enters your blood stream, lymphatic system, organs and cells. Bacteria, parasites, viruses, fungi, heavy metals, and chemicals in your blood stream will end up in your cells and organs, and if not removed can cause a clogged up, lymphatic system.

The key to healthy, holistic living is to limit your exposure to harmful contaminants and toxins, and to have a system in place for their regular removal. Otherwise, they will overwhelm you, your health and immune system will be compromised, and the road to pain free health will take a lot longer.

QUALITY OF THE ESSENTIAL OIL

Before buying essential oil, check the quality, and the reputation of the company manufacturing them. Check the essential oil purity, including the distillation method used, and whether there could be dilution with a cheap filler. A lower grade essential oil can be used for vaporization and breathing in, broadly applied within a room or home, but not for topical or internal use, and especially not on the young, pregnant, or those with compromised immune systems. Always

29

select the highest-grade essential oil that you can afford, as a little goes a long way. If you plan to take the essential oil internally, then use only the highest quality essential oil from a company, with an undisputed track record.

CHOOSING AN ESSENTIAL OIL

Essential oils have many different properties. Some assist the blood circulatory system, others work on the lymphatic system, others kill fungal spores, and others kill various strains of bacteria.

You may have a specific health, or living environment condition that would benefit from a different combination of essential oil, but those listed below have properties that neutralize most common types of bacteria, viruses, and fungi, and stimulate your immune system to cleanse your cells, organs, blood, and lymphatic fluids:

- Clove
- Lavender
- Lemon Grass
- Cinnamon
- Frankincense
- Myrrh
- Tea Tree
- Lemon
- Oregano
- Hyssop

VAPORIZATION

The easiest way to induce the health benefits of essential oil is to vaporize them. Place several drops of essential oil with some water into a vaporizing device, the simplest type is ceramic with a small candle as the heat source. The vapors neutralize any contaminants that are in the air you are breathing, such as viruses, fungi, and bacteria; and have a therapeutic effect on you. It is a good idea to keep a window open when vaporizing the essential oil so that you don't become overpowered by the smell. If the smell becomes too strong, then turn off the vaporizing device until the air clears.

Different members of the household, including your pets may prefer different fragrances, or they may have an aversion to some, and this needs to be taken into consideration when vaporizing essential oil.

Mixing essential oil for vaporizing will bring about the greatest concentrated benefit to you, because it may only be in your home, when you can use them, after a day in the office sitting in a building with sealed windows, and reticulated air. Take advantage of breathing in outside air whenever the air quality is good, because in many cities the air quality is poor, to very poor.

Place a few drops of each essential oil into the vaporizing device with water, using a maximum of three. Rotate daily the essential oil combinations vaporized, so that the different properties of each respective essential oil can be realized.

Try to mix essential oils that complement each other in fragrance, so that there are not too many objections from the household. Some fragrance combinations are more popular than others. The overall objective is to improve your household's health, not to make the home more fragrant, even though this is one of the benefits.

TOPICAL APPLICATION

During sleep time, your body repairs itself, your cells detoxify, and rejuvenate. For topical application, less is better, do a small patch test first on your skin to be certain that your body can tolerate the single, or combination of essential oil. Be aware that essential oil can have a heating effect, and for topical application, should be further diluted with a carrier oil such as coconut, or almond oil.

Due to the complementary properties, a blend of essential oil of typically three or four types, such as a sleep or relaxation mix, rather than a single essential oil should have a less intense, but a more effective remedial effect on your body.

Essential oil can be applied anywhere on your body. For maximum results, apply the essential oil to the soles of your feet due to the large number of sweat pores and blood vessels, and apply to the armpits, neck, and groin (the region between the abdomen and thighs) due to the high concentration of lymph nodes.

INTERNAL USE

For the consumption of an essential oil, the purity is critical, and limit the amount taken. Consume only a few drops, of only one type, of good quality, high grade essential oil in a glass of warm water in a day. Only use one essential oil type for a period of time, as you need to monitor your health benefits, and take regular breaks. The essential oil types that help improve your digestion, and breathing are frankincense, myrrh, and clove and they have anti-bacterial, fungal and parasitic properties.

The first essential oil to use is frankincense, as it helps significantly with digestive problems due to consuming food, and water contaminated with bacteria. The symptoms of acid reflux, bloating, fullness, and inability to digest food; due to the proliferation of gram-negative Helicobacter pylori in the stomach and small intestine can improve.

Myrrh essential oil is useful as a gateway essential oil, and can be used in rotation with frankincense essential oil. Take precautions if you are also on high blood pressure medications, or have a problem managing your blood sugar levels.

When your digestive issues are under control, switch to using clove essential oil, as it can help with reducing the symptoms associated with sinusitis, respiratory problems, and digestion. Clove essential oil can remove the biofilms that provide protection to bacteria, including antibiotic resistant gram-positive bacteria. Take precautions if you have high blood pressure, or take blood thinning medications as clove essential oil has its own natural properties.

CHAPTER TEN

DETOX STEP 6: PURE FRUIT SYRUPS, HERBAL AND BOTANICAL TONICS

How to use pure fruit syrups, herbal and botanical tonics of the TEN STEPS TO DETOX YOU – Detox Your Body And Feel Rejuvenated – Step Six.

If you are feeling unwell from a virus or bacteria, choose only one remedy to take internally, as too many different remedies taken at the same time could result in you getting a headache, and possibly vomiting. This maybe a faster removal of toxins, but pacing is also important in ensuring that you don't feel worse than when you started the detoxification process.

PURE FRUIT SYRUPS

Pure fruit syrups have been used for hundreds of years to provide vitamin C during the winter seasons, and are mostly taken as a cordial. Pure fruit syrups are an easy method for you to use to get your daily vitamin C, when your digestive system may not have the ability to break down a tablet, or capsule. It is also easy to replace soft drinks, and sugary cordials with pure fruit syrups in your household. Some options are black current, lemon, pomegranate and raspberry, but there are others to suit your taste.

HERBAL AND BOTANICAL TONICS

Herbal and botanical tonics are taken internally and can be purchased from most health food shops or chemists. Typically, a traditional botanical recipe is used. Swedish Bitters combines at least

33

11 herbs and Angelica root, for example. The purpose of these herbal and botanical tonics is to stimulate your digestive system, stimulating your liver for the production of bile, gallbladder in the release of bile, and spleen for the better cleansing of your blood. With improvement in your stomach acid, holistic improvement is experienced across the digestive system in eliminating various causes of illness. These tonics can help provide relief of colic in infants, and bloating in adults that are due to a poor digestive system.

Olive leaf extract tonic in liquid form is effective in assisting you to eliminate viruses. There are good quality Australian olive leaf extract tonics available, and the tonic is taken a few tablespoons at a time. Making a strong olive leaf tea is not as effective in riding the body of viruses, as the more concentrated tonic.

CHAPTER ELEVEN

DETOX STEP 7: CHARCOAL

How to use charcoal of the TEN STEPS TO DETOX YOU – Detox Your Body And Feel Rejuvenated – Step Seven.

Charcoal tablets are an important item to keep in your first aid kit, as they can save you from needing to visit a doctor's clinic or hospital.

Should you eat contaminated food, drink contaminated water, experience chemical or heavy metal exposure, and have mild symptoms, then charcoal tablets can be used to bind to these toxins. Allowing you to eliminate these toxins from your body, through the digestive system. The alternative could be that your body keeps circulating these toxins and your feeling of illness perpetuates.

Charcoal tablets are also useful if you have a virus with symptoms of digestive discomfort, or nausea. The use of charcoal tablets under these circumstances benefits your overall digestive system, liver, and kidneys. Charcoal tablets should not be used every day, as charcoal will also bind to beneficial minerals, and nutrients that you have consumed, preventing absorption.

NATASHA DAVIS

CHAPTER TWELVE

DETOX STEP 8: IODINE AND COLLOIDAL SILVER

How to use iodine and colloidal silver of the TEN STEPS TO DETOX YOU – Detox Your Body And Feel Rejuvenated – Step Eight.

Iodine and colloidal silver have both been used prior to the advent of antibiotics for healing purposes.

IODINE
Iodine can be applied topically to wounds as it breaks down biofilms, eliminating bacteria and fungi without harm.

Potassium iodine in liquid form, when taken as a few drops in water, gives immediate relief from viruses. Consuming potassium iodine can improve iodine levels in the body, and support the function of the thyroid as part of the immune system. If you are required to spend time in an environment with some radiation exposure, and/or with air viruses such as flying commercially, then consuming a few drops of potassium iodine in water after landing, showering and washing your hair can improve the functioning of your immune system, and stave off a viral infection.

COLLOIDAL SILVER
Colloidal silver is taken internally, a few tablespoons at one time. Monitor your body's ability to take the dosage of colloidal silver and adjust upwards, if you are not experiencing negative detox effects from the elimination of toxins such as headache and nausea. Before purchasing colloidal silver, make sure that it is good quality because besides the taste, the liquid is clear, so quality is hard to determine. Colloidal silver works by attaching itself to viruses and bacteria

(including antibiotic resistant) in the body, allowing you to eliminate them. Colloidal silver is useful in removing bacteria in hard to reach locations such as the sinuses, internal ear, and the digestive system.

CHAPTER THIRTEEN

DETOX STEP 9: REASSESS YOUR FRIENDSHIP CIRCLE AND HOBBIES

Reassess your friendship circle and hobbies of the TEN STEPS TO DETOX YOU – Detox Your Body And Feel Rejuvenated – Step Nine.

Negative energy, and toxicity from other people can reduce your happiness. These people act like energy thieves stealing your positive energy, replacing it with their negative energy, and ultimately draining you. These negative people could be those closest to you. People you've known all your life. They use you as an energy replenishment source, and can prove to be extra-ordinarily difficult to remove from your life.

YOUR FRIENDSHIP CIRCLE

Start with changing your focus, from your friendship circle, to you. Make time for yourself by doing what is important for you, and these activities feed your positive energy, sense of worth, and happiness. Set boundaries for yourself, and protect these boundaries. Perseverance is important, as you will experience negative reactions directed towards you, when you enforce your boundaries. These negative people will be very unhappy that you are not spending your most valuable resource, which is your time, doing emotional and physical work for them. This work can include doing their personal chores, office work, spending your money on them, being an outlet for their extensive problems, and conflicts that they create with everyone that crosses their path. These negative people may also

39

start calling you unhappy and negative, but this is just projection of their negative emotions onto you.

By allocating more time for yourself, you will discover more about yourself and ways you want to spend your time that provide you with more value. Along this journey, you will meet new people, some you may want to keep as long-term friends, and others you will clearly see as people with a lot of negativity, that they want you to absorb for them. This is the process of developing your own self-worth, and these personal qualities will protect you from seeking refuge in habits (such as gambling, excessive drinking, drug use including prescription drugs), and friends that manipulate and control you. The goal is to demonstrate personal leadership. To not be led by others, and to not need to control, and manipulate others around you.

YOUR HOBBIES

Your hobbies should add value to your life. If you are doing these hobbies only because they are habitual, or you get to socialize with a group of people that otherwise would not make time for you, then you have better opportunities elsewhere.

A hobby can cost you a lot of time and money, and there should be a return on this investment. These are extra-ordinary joy, skills to earn you income, and better life coping skills of improvements to your self-control and resiliency, so you can avoid falling into emergency financial and health situations.

CHAPTER FOURTEEN

DETOX STEP 10: REASSESS YOUR FINANCIAL OUTFLOWS AND TIME-CONSUMING RESPONSIBILITIES

Reassess your financial outflows and time-consuming responsibilities of the TEN STEPS TO DETOX YOU – Detox Your Body And Feel Rejuvenated – Step Ten.

The act of simplifying your life can reduce your internal, toxic load enormously. It is known that significant anxiety is caused from personal financial distress, and trying to meet financial obligations. Just as having many personal relationship obligations causes anxiety, the same results from having complicated financial arrangements that take up your time. The easiest starting point is to reduce your expenses.

FINANCIAL OUTFLOWS
Some examples of complicated financial arrangements include having several bank accounts and credit cards, government fees, utilities, home rent or mortgage, rent of cars and furniture, insurances, school fees, hospital fees, business debts, and other accumulated financial debts.

Do you need the latest gadget, car, fashion accessory?

41

Do you find that you didn't get the expected satisfaction from spending all that time to find, buy and learn how to use stuff you were convinced you needed?

Is your home crowded with possessions in various states of deterioration?

Make an assessment of how you can reduce your general outgoing costs in relation to housing, utilities, food, transport, education, medical, and entertainment.

TAKE STOCK OF WHAT YOU HAVE

Hold off on buying anything new until you know what you actually want, and what will be useful to you in the near future. The result is that you will achieve clarity on what items you really want surrounding you daily, and taking up your time in needing to be cleaned, and maintained.

Start by going shopping in your home, clean out and throw out stuff you haven't been using. Play a game that involves looking through the items in your house that haven't been used recently, or at all, and try to find a way to use them, as a starting point, choose three items.

The options for the item are to use as originally intended or repurpose the item. If you can't come up with any ideas, then put the item aside for a few weeks, and if you still don't have any ideas on what to do with the item, then give it away.

The result of this approach is wearing clothes and shoes that haven't been worn much, finding that clothes and shoes have deteriorated from the humidity, and can no longer be worn, finding that clothes and shoes no longer fit your comfort requirements, shape and lifestyle needs, including your hobbies.

Going through fabric collections in the house including tablecloths, bed spreads, and curtains and making new items of clothing and bags. Making items of furniture out of existing furniture you own, and simple crafts such as book marks.

These activities can be a fun, and cost-effective way to spend time together for families and friends.

TIME NEEDED FOR CLEANING AND MAINTENANCE

Have you ever kept an item for a rainy day?

Only, to find out later that the item deteriorated with age, or became afflicted with rust, mold, or water damage.

If you are not using the item now, or plan to use the item in the near future due to household needs, or seasonal use, and the item is in good condition, then the best option is to sell the item now to maximize the sale price you can receive.

On reducing your expenses, calculate, and make an assessment, of whether it is cheaper for you to use public transport, and hire a car when needed, instead of buying and maintaining a car. Include in this calculation the need to have an emergency vehicle taking into account the factors of where you live, such as remoteness, potential for natural disasters and civil unrest, and the need to have an emergency vehicle due health issues of the household.

Eat foods that are simple, nutrient filled, uncomplicated to make, and easy to digest. That fancy, expensive meal may just give you digestive issues, and health issues. If you have suffered from food poisoning in the past, then your own home cooking is the best way to avoid future food poisoning.

REMOVE OBLIGATIONS FROM YOUR LIFE

Draw up a list of activities that you enjoy doing, and make sure that you have time to do these activities. You will need to drop some activities you are currently doing, release some friends from your friendship circle, and all that this means is that you are growing as a person. Because to stop growing means, that your body, and mind will weaken, and you will run out of time to do everything you wanted to do during your life.

NATASHA DAVIS

CHAPTER FIFTEEN

NEXT STEPS

Have you ever wondered what makes some people old, and some people young when not taking into consideration their physical age?

Why a 35-year-old who is settled into a routine, can seem boring, without any desire to experience new interests, but an 85-year-old is not, and vice versa?

LIFE PLAN
Is the secret, just simply having a life plan?

Having a reason to get up every day, and to do a bit more, than you did yesterday?

The 'Template For Your Life Plan' (in the next chapter) allows you to prioritize, and organize your time over a five-year horizon so that you achieve your life keystones.

LIFE CHALLENGES
Achieving your life plan can be difficult when you don't feel well, your body aches all over, there seems to be no identifiable cause, or you are diagnosed with a new, rare disease. You may have additional challenges due to the circumstances of your life from accidents, war, natural disasters, hazardous chemicals, radiation, fungi, and other contaminated environments. Achieving, and maintaining good health for yourself, and your household is extremely important, and it is a key component of your life plan. You will experience significant financial, emotional, and physical costs if you are not in good health.

DETOX SYSTEM
TEN STEPS TO DETOX YOU can help you wind back any damage done to your physical body. The body is amazing in its ability

to heal itself, it is an extremely complicated system, and what works for person A, will not work for person B, because lifestyle choices have been different over the course of a person's life. Taking your own personalized detox steps, monitoring, and assessing how you feel in relation to these actions is the best path to follow.

NEXT STEPS

TEN STEPS TO DETOX YOU gives you a starting point to take more control over your life, and the 'Template For Your Life Plan' aids you in living a more purposeful life.

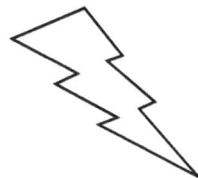

Blue Skies and Cloudy Mornings

Patchwork quilt skies of blue and white
Rainclouds in the distant sky
Hot coffee in my favorite mug
Reminds me of times of old.

Friends come past and say hello
Whispering stories of times of old
Memories of love and happiness
Down pours and sadness.

Sunlight shines through the new dreams of color
Dew glistens on the grass
Kaleidoscope of potential
Horizons bring forward the new.

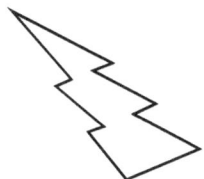

NATASHA DAVIS

CHAPTER SIXTEEN

TEMPLATE FOR YOUR LIFE PLAN

The 'Template for Your Life Plan' is a guide that you can fill in using the next five years as the timeline.

Your life plan can help you identify what is important to you, so that these goals and activities are prioritized.

Your life plan can help you to better allocate and prioritize your time.

Your life plan can also make sure you take actions to improve your resiliency to unplanned events, to do the tasks that will improve your life, but are not fun, or enjoyable to do.

HOW TO FILL IN THE TEMPLATE FOR YOUR LIFE PLAN

➤ Use a five-year timeline.

➤ **Life Plan** box – insert your name in front of Life Plan to claim responsibility.

➤ **Health and Happiness** box – list items such as overall health, fitness activities etc.

➤ **Career** box – list items such as promotion, career enhancement, further study, self-employed etc.

- ➢ **Love** box – list items such as protection: physical, emotional, spiritual etc.

- ➢ **Connectivity** box – list items such as community, family, friends, pets etc.

- ➢ Then you have your **Special Project Areas** on what you want to achieve over the next 5 years.

- ➢ **Asset Management** box – list house, cash, pension etc.

- ➢ **Rewards** box – list incomes, recognition for achievements/doing good work etc.

- ➢ **Energy Flows** box – list balance creating activities such as hobbies, sleep, exercise etc.

- ➢ **Development Activities** box – list sharing information, harmonizing actions, another people's welfare.

TEN STEPS TO DETOX YOU

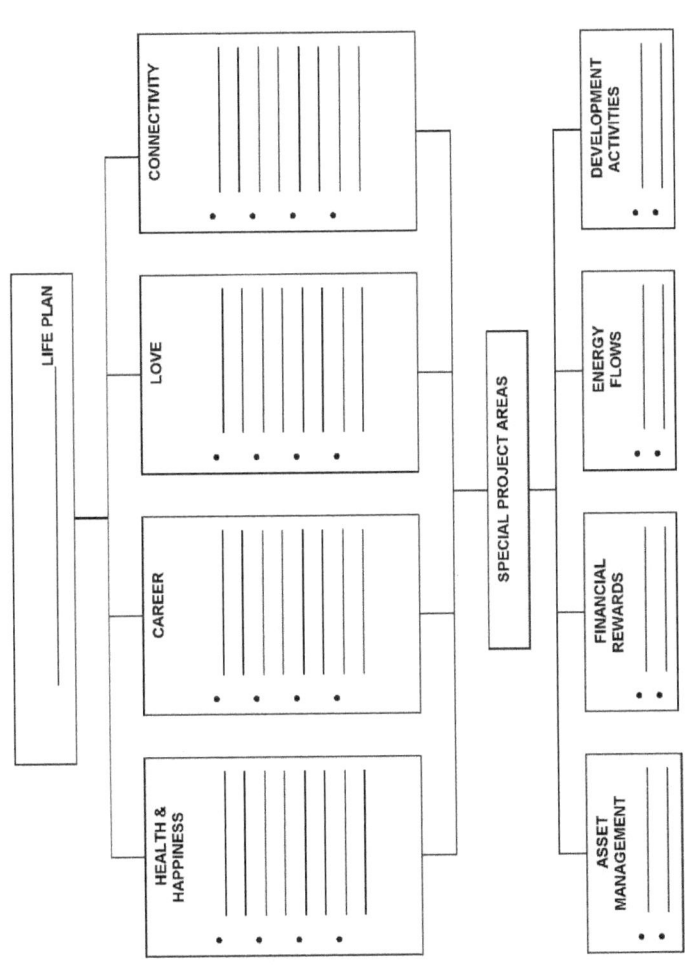